Living with Mental Illnesses
for the diagnosed and those who love you

By Kimberly M Schouppe

Dedication

I dedicate this book to anyone out there struggling with any form of mental illness. You are amazing, you are loved, and you got this! Never give up, no matter how hard it gets, keep pushing forward! You are a warrior! You got this!

Foreward

Are you struggling with mental illness(es)? If so, you are not alone. Each year, there are approximately 5% of adults 18 and over diagnosed with a form of mental illness, that means it is equivalent to approximately 43.8 million people diagnosed. In the US, about 14.4 percent have one mental disorder, and about 5.8 percent have two disorders, and about 6 percent have 3 or more disorders. And it is said that approximately 5.3 million adults 18 and over are diagnosed with bipolar disorder. It is estimated that 51% of these individuals go untreated each year. I want you to know, no matter who you are or what your diagnoses is, there is always help out there for you. There are doctors, hospitals, therapists, and organizations that can help get you diagnosed and get you on the right medications for your diagnoses. You are not alone. There are also groups out there that you can meet with or online via social media where you discuss your diagnoses in a warm and open manner with no judgement. In this book, I will be sharing with you my journey of being diagnosed with bipolar 2 disorder, Anxiety, and Depression. I will share with you my symptoms, thoughts, and feelings leading up to being diagnosed and the medication process. I hope that you find this helpful and that it helps you to get your own diagnoses and to get the strength and courage to push forward and not let these illnesses rule your life. Bless you all, love and light to you. May you be prosperous in all your endeavors.

Acknowledgements

First and foremost, I would like to thank my parents Virginia Booth and Brian Schouppe for always teaching me to be strong, to never give up, and to always follow my heart and dreams. For always supporting me and helping me in any way they could from a baby until now. Thank you, mom and dad, I love you. I would also like to acknowledge my grandmothers who are no longer with us on this earth, but are with us in spirit; Sylvia Schouppe and Mildred Booth, gone but never forgotten. I love and miss you both more than words can say, thank you both so much for being such strong and loving women and positive role models. Also want to thank Jessica L Weishuhn gone but never forgotten, I am so lucky that I got to know and be friends with you. And I hope you are watching over us and my daughter Jessica, your namesake. Next, I would like to thank my sister Kaitlyn Schouppe, my brother Josh Smith, and my boyfriend George Barriero. And to my children Dominic Rivera and Jessica Barreiro; mommy loves you so much. You are the reasons I keep going even when I feel like giving up. You are the greatest blessings I have ever recieved. And to my aunts, uncles, cousins, and my many friends! I love you all!! And I thank you all so much for being a part of my life and for loving and accepting me for who I am. You have all been by my side and when I needed you the most. You all mean the world to me.

"Don't stop believin, hold on to that feelin"
Steve Perry from Journey...

Chapter 1. My early life

It all started in my early teenage years when I was 15 years old, I was your average kid, you know the type; hardly any friends, constantly picked on and made fun of for various reasons. The depressed but didn't show it kid. The one who put up an emotional front so no one would see all the emotional and mental pain I was going through. I had ok grades and was doing ok until Wednesday February 13th 2002, when my world came to a grinding halt, I had lost my grandmother Syliva Irene Schouppe. To say I was devastated is an understatement, I felt as though my world came crashing down and that my heart was ripped out of my chest, stuffed in a blender and pureed. My dad's brother who was my Uncle Terry Schouppe (also deceased) and his wife sped into our driveway and ran in our house, as my mom was about to yell at him about the way he flew into our driveway and just came in the house; he pulled her aside and gave her the news: "mom is gone" he said to her. His wife was the one to tell me. I'll never forget those horrible words: "Grandma Schouppe is gone, she passed away in her sleep". I was shocked, I kicked a hole in our hallway wall. I started crying and freaked out! I was so angry and sad that she was gone. I was angry and lashed out at everyone, I was very depressed and always crying. My grades started slipping a lot. The school told my mom about a place in Stroudsburg called MHMR Services. It was help for individuals with mental illness and behavioral problems. So, she ended up taking me there for an evaluation and services for my behavior. I had the evaluation done and they said there was a possibility of depression, anxiety and bipolar disorder and I needed a more thorough psych evaluation, which I refused. I had a worker named Jamie who came to our house to sit and talk with me and she also took me out places such as the library or the mall for talks and therapy. I also ended up having to go to summer school to make up the classes that I failed. In the years following, I became increasingly depressed and angry. I started to not listen to my parents or any adult really. I started going and staying out whenever I wanted to, not calling or coming home for days. Only came home when I felt like it. I started cutting when I was about 16. I started taking pills at 17 and drinking. At the age of 18, I had taken a lot of pills and also drank quite a bit at the same time. It scared me when I woke up the next morning and was yelled at by a friend who told me she stayed up all night long watching me to make sure I was breathing. I decided then that I was going to stop taking the pills, and stop drinking and cutting. I stopped it all by myself, no rehab, all on my own at 18. My behaviors were still getting worse as I got older. I moved out at 18, was in an on and off relationship, had my first child at 22 and turned 23 a week later. I suffered through severe post-partum depression. My OB/GYN put me on the antidepressant Zoloft which, as it turned out, I have an allergy to. My relationship with my son's father completely ended when my son turned 1 year old. But thankfully I had my parents there to help me as well as my grandmother Millie. I also was on TANF and WIC which helped a lot as well. But on December 15th, 2011. Things once again changed. That was the day my grandmother Mildred Louise Booth passed away. It was yet again another devastating blow. But I'm thankful my son got to spend 2 years with her and got to love her and know her love for him. He absolutely loved going to her house. One of his favorite things to do was play with her cow vacuum cover. He always got so sad when wehad to leave. He adored her so much. And when she passed he was still little, he was only 2 years old, and I'm glad that he didn't know what was going on and wasn't sad like we were when she passed. He is older now, 11. He understands now what death is and srill surprises me with how smart he is. Jessica is now 8 years old and she is so smart and understands so much just like her brother.

Chapter 2. Life goes on

After my grandmother Millie passed, we moved to Easton PA. While there I switched my TANF and WIC from Monroe County to Northampton County and continued going to their program at the Career Link in Easton. While living in Easton, I met my Boyfriend George. We have been together almost 10 years now, and we have a beautiful daughter Jessica. Jessica is named after a friend of mine who passed away after a car accident. Her name was Jessica Lynn Weishuhn. I took her death very hard because we were childhood friends. I'm glad she has a namesake, and I'm glad it is my daughter. I took my daughter for the first time to meet Jess's mom on Easter. It was a beautiful moment although, to be perfectly honest, I was terrified that it would be too hard and sad on her mom Gabby. But it was beautiful, her mom fell in love with her. She hugged me and thanked me for giving their family such a beautiful gift, what was this gift you may be wondering? Well, the gift was that their beloved Jess had a namesake. After about a year or so we moved back to the Poconos, back to Canadensis. In 2013 I could no longer take the constant depressed, anxious, and scary mood swings I was constantly going through. So, what did I do? I went back to MHMR in Stroudsburg and was seen by a Psychologist and FINALLY got a diagnosis... and that diagnosis was Generalized Anxiety Disorder, and Bipolar 2 Disorder with Bipolar Aggression. What does that mean? Well, basically it means that I have anxiety and bipolar disorder with depression and aggressive tendencies. This means that my form of bipolar disorder has more depressive and aggressive lows than manic highs. This means that my mood swings could be more dangerous with very aggressive and possibly violent lashing out and being very short tempered to those around me including those I love and care about. It also means that very depressed states could result in loss of appetite, interest, suicide or attempts, and possible hospitalization especially when not on medication. After being properly diagnosed, I was finally being properly treated. I was put on medications and seeing a psychologist and a therapist. Let me tell you, those medications are a big help, and seeing a therapist is a wonderful way to vent your thoughts and feelings without judgement and fear. They offer so many good suggestions on coping skills such as journaling, exercising, etc. They may also suggest anger management to help you deal with any rage you may have due to your illness. I highly suggest this. They are there to hlep you, not judge you, they genuinely care about your health and well being and safety.

Chapter 3. Medication

So, after being properly diagnosed, I was put on a mood stabilizer and a medication for my anxiety. I also saw a therapist about once a week. And believe me when I say that seeing a therapist to vent and talk to about your thoughts and feelings without being judged, is an awesome feeling! It's like a weight has been lifted and finally feeling free. At first, I was put on 450 mg of Lithium and 25 mg of Atarax. I personally felt that was too high of a dosage and I did not want to take the Lithium at all. Why? Well before I could even start the Lithium, I had to have bloodwork done and an EKG to make sure my heart was strong enough to take the medication. Then once I started taking the medication, I would have to go for routine bloodwork to make sure my levels were good. I didn't want to have to go through that. So, I ended up once again moving. I got a new family doctor and we went over my diagnoses and medications. When we got to the Lithium, we both agreed it was too much and I was then put on Lamictal. Started off at 25 mg for a week, then 50, until I was increased to 100 mg. She kept my Atarax at the same dosage. The medications have been very helpful and work great for me. They help with the anxiety and severity and frequency of my mood swings, they have me feeling like a "normal" person. Without proper medication and treatment mental illnesses can be very dangerous to the person with the illness and those around them. Many can have explosive violent fits of rage, when this happens the person will not only be a danger to themself, but to others around them. People who are not treated can end up in jail when in reality they should be hospitalized and evaluated and treated. These people do not mean to cause harm to themselves or anyone else. There are different types of medications depending on the illness or disorder. There are mood stabilizers, antidepressants, antipsychotics, antianxiety, your Dr will determine which of these medications you will need and which brand and dosage. If you are prescribed a medication be sure to take it as directed and at the same time everyday. Do not skip doses, and do not go off your medication without your Dr kmowing. Going off your meds can have dangerous side effects such as rage, violence toward others, and sometimes psychosis that ends in suicide. The medications are designed to help the chemical imbalance in the brain, going off your meds and too fast will mess the imbalance up more and faster. PLEASE keep a medication schedule, make a reminder. If you have a hard time, have a friend or family member make the schedule for you and administer your medication to you. It is important not to take any more than the Dr says to take as this can lead to accidental or purposeful overdose. If you have any side effects or allergies to your medication you need to immediately report this to your Dr to have your meds changed. Some side effects and allergies are as follows: dry mouth, nausea, voimiting, diarreah, rash, swelling of face and/or tongue or throat. Any of these need to be roported immediately as some can be severe and life threatening.

Chapter 4. Family and Relationships

Dealing with family members and trying to have a relationship with someone who has bipolar disorder or any other mental illness or disorder can be very hard and sometimes impossible. As a person with bipolar disorder myself, we often times get afraid no one will love us and want to genuinely be with us so we tend to push people away and shut them out, which then causes us depression. Dealing with a loved one with a mental illness or disorder is no walk in the park, it's not sunshine and rainbows. It is VERY HARD, AND VERY DIFFICULT. But it can also be VERY GOOD AND WONDERFUL when the loved one is getting proper treatment, proper medications at the right dosage, and is cooperating and talking with their team of psychologist and therapist and continues to take the meds. I'm not going to lie or sugarcoat things, it does take a lot of patience and understanding your loved one's diagnosis. I know, I'm bipolar myself. We need a lot of reassurance that you are here for us and that you are not going to abandon us when we need you. We need you to be patient with us during our manic or low episodes. We need you to understand that it is not our fault that we act the way we do. We need you. Point blank period, we need you. You are our family, a girlfriend, boyfriend, husband, or wife. We need you to be there at our worst as well as our best to cheer us on and tell us to keep pushing and never give up. For a lot of people with bipolar disorder or any for of menatl illness , they don't have that kind of support system and often turn to drug and alcohol addiction and it often ends up sadly in an accidental overdose, or suicide. You as a care giver need to watch for the signs of addiction, If you do notice it you need to act accordingly and bring it to their attention that you are very concerned. You may need to have them confined to a treatment center until they have gotten through withdrawl and are on the right medication and treatment plan. Suggest that they make you the power of attorney in case anything were to happen to them, a life insurance policy to help their loved ones if and when they pass on which can help give them peace of mind. Anything can happen from a severe allergy, accidental overdose, or suicide. Have a will drawn up as well. Now the reason I am saying to do all this is in case of a medical emergency that reults in death. ***It is no way meant t***o make them or the family worried in any way, it is just to have things in place in case anything happened to them. You just want to reassure them all will be taken care of.

Chapter 5. Befriending a person with a Mental Illness

When you first meet someone with bipolar disorder, or depression, etc. You will at first think we are a regular average person. But when we tell you we have a mental illness and you finally see the symptoms and episodes we have, please don't drop us like a bad habit. And please DO NOT TREAT US ANY DIFFERENTLY! We don't like being treated any differently than you would treat other friends, and we don't like being treated like we are a bother or like we are stupid. We don't like being treated like children either. We have thoughts and feelings too. Treat us the same as you would anyone else. If you are going to be friends with someone who has a ment l illness please do some research about our illness, please try to understand what we go through on a daily basis and why it happens. And when you introduce us to your other friends or to your family please do not go "hey this is so and so, and he/she has some brain issues" not only is that a very mean thing to say, but it can trigger us into an episode that will have us feeling bad and embarrassed. Don't do that. Introduce us like you would anyone else. Please do not talk behind our backs, we just like anyone else can and will hear about it and that hurts us like it would anyone else. And that can send us into a very deep depression and some never make it out and it ends up in suicide for a lot of people. And please do not call us crazy people or retarded people, it is offensive and poor choice of words. It i very degrading and we feel it is cruel and that we are not wanted. treat us with love, care, and respect. We are not bad people, we are people who just so happen to have an illness that is not our fault. We did NOT ask for or choose to have these illnesses or disorders. But, they are here to stay, they are for life. So buckle up for a wild and crazy ride.

Chapter 6. Family History

Ok, now let's talk about family history...

So, first and foremost folks; you need to understand that these illnesses are hereditary. They can and do pass down from family member to family member. So, let's say, that mom has no illness but dad does, what does this mean for their child? It means that there is a chance that later on in life it could be discovered that the child could have an illness as well. And when they have children of their own it could be passed down the line. If you suspect that you or your child may have a mental illness it is important to be evaluated, but, be aware that they can only evaluate a child when the child is old enough. They will most likely evaluate and treat around the age of 5. When being evaluated by a psychologist or doctor for a mental illness they will ask you about family history. Family history of what exactly? Well, a family history of mental illness, cancer, blood pressure, cholesterol, etc. It is extremely important to answer those questions truthfully to the best of your ability, if you need to you can ask about family history before you go to your appointment or bring a family member with you who can answer what you don't know. Any information you don't know or intentionally leave out can lead to problems being treated properly. You need to be open and fully transparent when giving family history, they are there to help you not judge you. They need to know these things so that they know what tests to order before you start on a medication. This will help you in the long run to prevent certain side effects and reduce the risk of any allergies.

Chapter 7. How to tell people you have a Mental Illness

When it comes to telling others that you have a mental illness it can be scary and hard. Don't let it be that way. Honesty and communication are key. Be open and honest. Sit whoever you are telling down and tell them that you would like to tell them something and that you will explain things after and answer any questions they may have afterward. Start by telling them that you were seen by a doctor, tell them it was a psychologist. Explain that you are ok and there is no need to worry. Tell them that you were diagnosed with a disorder and that you will be fine and you will be on medication and you will be seeing a therapist as well as your psych Doctor as part of your treatment plan. Tell them you are fine and that you will explain in further detail about your disorder.Do not be afraid to tell your employer or potential employer as they can not refuse to hire you or fire you for your diangosis because that would be dicrimination and could turn into a lawsuit which they don't want. Answer any questions they have to the best of your ability and suggest that if they would like to, they can do research about it online. Tell them, that by them doing research and understanding what you are or will go through they are being supportive and helpful in a big and positive way and that you appreciate them for doing so. Let them know that they are a big part of your treatment just by doing research, accompanying you to appointments, and by being a listening ear and a shoulder to cry and lean on. Just by being supportive, and sticking by someone with a mental illness can and has saved lives. So, please if you are someone who was told by your family member, friend, husband, wife, girlfriend, or boyfriend has a mental illness, please stay by their side. They will need you more than you know. You will be one of the biggest parts of their support and treatment. Learn all you can and try to understand the illness and please understand that certain behaviors are not their fault. Understand that is an illness that no one asked to have. They are normal people too, they just have an illness that they are treating as best as they can.

Chapter 8. *What is Mental Illness?*

A mental Illness is classified as a wide range of conditions that affect the mood, thinking, and behavior of a person. It is a chemical imbalance in the human brain that causes a multitude of mental illnesses such as depression, and bipolar disorder. Some other examples would be anxiety disorder, and Schizophrenia. There are many types of mental illnesses. Some examples are obsessive compulsive disorder, post-traumatic stress disorder, panic disorder, eating disorders, personality disorders etc. It is extremely important that you follow you doctor's instuctions and treatment plan they have put together for you after you have been diagnosed. It is also extremely important as a friend, family member, or care giver that you also follow the diagnosed person's treatment plan exactly. It would also be important and beneficial for you as the friend, family member, or care giver to research the diagnosis. Researching the illnes is very beneficial to you because you will get a better understanding of the illness, medications, hospitializations etc. It is important to make a note of medications being taken, the exact dosage and mg, the phone numbers of all doctors the patient sees, and all the phone numbers for psych hospitals and crisis lines. You should also know the full name, age, and date of birth of the patient for emergency reasons and it may also be good to know the blood type as well. The more information about the diagnosed is very beneficial and important to their overall health, and their safety as well as the safety of others around them. You need to understand that if an emergency arises and you need to call someone and that it is for the best. It is not a punishment; it is for their own good and for the good of those around. You are not being mean or being the bad guy, you are doing your job and the right thing for them as a friend, family member, or care giver. You may feel horrible at first, but please don't! Please do not pity or feel bad for us. If anything, we would be grateful to you for caring enough to help us even if we don't show it or tell you at first. At first, we may be angry, sad, and resentful that you called and had us transported to a facility designed to help us. But, after a while some will be grateful and glad you helped, and some won't, some may stay resentful and angry for a longer period of time, some for life. But just know you did nothing wrong; you did what you were supposed to do, you did the right thing. You stepped up and intervened to make sure the patient and those around them were safe. Wonderful job, keep up the good work, they will appreciate you for all your love, support, and help in making difficult decisions.

Chapter 9. Parenting and Mental Illness

Another challenge while having a mental illness or disorder is parenting. You worry what if you pass it on to your child? What if your child passes it on to their children etc. Or your child may have inherited a mental illness or disorder from someone else in the family and you may be wondering what will happen to them? How do you and your child deal with the illness? Well, the answer to those questions is simple: DO NOT PANIC. That's right, do not panic. Panicking only makes the situation worse for everyone. Simply go see a professional for an evaluation, get a diagnosis,ge on a treatment plan, and take any medications as prescribed and recommended. Do not treat your child any differently. Make them comfortable with the diagnosis and tell them it's ok. Tell them they are just like everyone else. If they feel bad and talk bad about themselves it is YOUR JOB to talk to them and build up their self-esteem and help them build up their confidence and self-worth. Tell them it's ok to feel things, but not to let it take over them. Have them if they are old enough to write and keep a well documented journal of their thoughts and feelingsthat may come with their illness. Have them think of a hobby they like such as writing, painting, walking, etc to help them if they feel bad or have an episode, it will help keep them calm and take their mind off of what is going on. Go to the park, bike ride, or go swimming with them. For a parent with a mental illness or disorder it can be very scary not knowing if your child will inherit your illness or disorder. You need to just relax and take it one day at a time. If one day your child exhibits some of the symptoms of an illness take them to a professional for an evaluation. But until then, relax, take care of your mental health. Follow your treatment plan, take your meds, and see your mental health team. Discuss any new or worsening symptoms. Keep your support team updated and make sure they know what to do to help you in case of a severe episode or crisis. Make sure they know about your diagnosis and symptoms, make sure they did their research on your illness or disorder. Keep a journal of your feelings, symptoms, mood swings, etc. Keep this to show your mental health team at each appointment. This can be very helpful and beneficial in your treatment plan. Remember, to always love and support any parent or child with any form of mental illness. It is no their fault, they did not ask for or choose it, and they just want to be loved and understood and not be treated any different. And let them be free to be themselves and express themselves. This is important as you don't want them to feel like they are being restricted. Also they may need special help in school such as special education, emotional support, a tss worker also known as a theraputic support specialst, and behavioral support. Always make sure the school nurse is aware of their special needs and medications.

Chapter 10. Pregnancy and Medication

Finding out you are pregnant is an exciting and special time! But if you have a mental illness it can be a scary time. You find out that you probably won't be able to take your medication(s) because of the risk of harmful birth defects or possible miscarriage. Some medications have been studied an known to cause a lot of different and severe birth defects and loss of pregnancy. As frightening as that may seem, you can talk to your Dr about other ways to continue to manage your illness while pregnant. Do not be discouraged about treatment and pregnancy, a lot of women have had happy, healthy pregnancies and delivered healthy babies. There are also mommy groups you could join on social media such as Facebook. Research them and if they appeal to you and are what you are looking for, you can join and talk about your problems and get some very good and helpful advice. I myself have joined mommy groups on social media and I absolutely love the other ladies in the groups. They are so supportive and offer a ton of good advice and solutions. I highly recommend joing one of these groups. There are also wonderful mental health groups on social media you could join to talk and vent about your mental health journey and struggles as well as your pregnancy.

Chapter 11. Getting a Diagnosis

If you feel you or a loved one is exhibiting signs or symptoms of a mental illness or disorder, the first step is to acknowledge it. It is important to acknowledge this because it means you are aware and can then seek out help. To seek out help means searching for the right kind of provider. Now to find the right provider you must first contact your insurance company. If you don't have insurance you can apply for state medical insurance through your local County Assistance Office. Or if it is an emergency you can go to the nearest local hospital and explain what is going on and the severity, they may admit you, evaluate you, and start you on medication. They can also help get you started on obtaining insurance to be able to continue treatment with a provider and to keep you on your medication. When you find the right provider, they will do a mental health evaluation which consists of a variety of questions about your symptoms and family history as well as your current health condition. Going to the Dr for your mental health is not a sign of weakness as some would make you believe. Going to the Dr for mental health is a good thing. It means you know that something is not right and you need help. For those who suspect a friend or member of your family has an illness or disorder, it is not wrong to ask them to see someone and for you to tell them that you will go with them for support. That is a good first step to helping them. It is a commendable effort on your part, it shows them that you care about and love them enough to help get them on a good road to treatment. Go with them to any appointment they want you to go to, ask questions, and do your research. Make sure your concern is genuine and true or else they may think you don't care and that you just want to get rid of them. Keep a well-documented journal of their actions and what they say for the Dr. This will helpthe Dr determine the plan and course of action and medication involved with the treatment plan.

Chapter 12. Emotional Support

Being emotionally supportive is a **_mus_**t in dealing with someone who has any form of mental illness or disorder. This shows them that you care. They need this more than you know. Often times, they feel scared and alone. They may feel like no one understands or cares about them and what they are going through. You need to show them that that is not the case. You need to ask questions, ask how they are doing, do they need anything. Go with them to appointments and ask the Dr questions. Make sure they keep their appointments, and make sure they are taking their medication. Being emotionally supportive means showing interest in their diagnosis and treatment. Showing interest and care in them and their feelings. It also means sitting with them through episodes, being a listening ear, and a shoulder to cry and lean on. Emotional support is knowing when to take them to the hospital when the episode is severe and they are a danger to themselves and others. It will be hard and scary but, in the end, you did the right and best thing for them. Always answer any calls or text messages asking for help, you must always assume they are serious whether they are or not. This builds trust between you. This shows them that you do indeed care and only want what is best for them.

Chapter 13. Coping Skills and Strategies

Some good coping skills would be journaling. Start a journal starting from when you got your diagnosis. Keep your journal well documented about all your thought and feelings, this will not only help you cope with your illness or disorder, but it can also help your treatment team to halp you better. How? Well by you keeping such a well written and documented journal full of all your thoughts and feelings this will help your Dr determine if you need a medication increase, decrease, or be swapped for another or to have another added. You could also start a blog or vlog to help others with mental illnesses or disorders. You could start a podcast as well. You can paint, go for walks and exercise, read, listen to calming music. Drawing is also a good coping strategy to use. If you can't think of any other strategies you can use, you can most certainly ask your Dr, counselor, or therapist for ideas and help.

Chapter 14. Celebrities with Mental Illness

Yes you read that right, even celebrities suffer from mental illnesses and disorders. Stars such as Demi Lovato, Michale Phelps, Robin Williams, Chester Bennington, Chrissy Teigen, Steve Young, Donny Osmond, Dan Reynolds, Daniel Radcliffe, and Leonardo Dicaprio just to name a few. The above stars mentioned suffer from ilnesses such as post partum depression, obsessive compulsive disorder, bipolar disorder, adhd, social anxiety disorder, clinical depression, and so many more. So, most likely, a celebrity hero of yours may also have a form of mental illness as well. And if they can get the help they need to live an ordinary life you can too. But unfortunately, for some it just becomes too much and leads to alcoholism, drug addiction, and suicide. Even the tars take medications to manage. Medications such as Lamictal aka Lamictogrine, Ataraox aka Hydroxozine, Depakote, Seroquel, Xanax, Lithium, Latuda, Abilify, Clozapine, Zyprexa, Zoloft, Wellbutrin, Aderall, Risperdall, etc. So never be ashamed to admit that you have an illness or disorder, the stars aren't ashamed of theirs.A lot of them actually want to help others in the world who suffer from mental health problems, that is amazing.

Chapter 15. Important Information

National Suicide Prevention Hotline: 1-800-273-8255

Depression help: www.psychiatry.org

Bipolar Help: www.helpguide.org

National Institute of Mental Health: www.nimh.nih.gov

You can also reach out to local mental health organizations, local hospitals, and your local county assistance office to apply for insurance. You can go to the office or fill out an application online. You will create a username and password if filling out the application online. You will need your social security card, driver's license or state issued ID, and any unpaid medical bills. Next, you will have an in person or phone interview with a case worker to determine if you are elligeable for insurance. Once approved you will receive information in the mail as well as your new insurance card. Then you will pick your providers, your new insurance will also include a phone number for mental and behavioral health.

Isnpirational Quotes

" What mental health needs is more sunlight, more candor, and more unashamed conversation" - Glenn Cose

" The ony journey, is the journey WITHIN" - Rainer Maria Rilke

" Just because you don't understand it, doesn't mean it isn't so" - Lemony Snicket, The Blank Book

" The problem with having probems is that someone always has it worse" -Tiffany Madison, Black and White

"Always remember, you do not have to struggle in silence, and alone; there are others out there going through the same things and are there to help you and understand you; you are all amazing warriors keep fighting" - Kimberly Marie Schouppe

Conclusion:

Always be a loving, supportive friend, family membe, or care giver. They need you. Always be calm especially in case of an emergency. Never panic because it only makes things worse. Talk to them, make them feel important and do not yell at or make them feel bad.

Never be afraid to reach out if you or someone you love is in need of desperate and immediate help. It is not a sign of weakness; you are not the bad guy. It shows that you are strong and that you love them and care for them. Always remember that no matter what, you are here for a reason, everyone has a purpose in life. You are amazing, special, and loved. You got this! You are a mental health warrior so keep on fighting, keep on pushing. Never be afraid to reach out and ask for help.

www.ingramcontent.com/pod-product-compliance
Lightning Source LLC
Chambersburg PA
CBHW030519220526
45464CB00006B/2869